ANSWERS TO THE 100 QUESTIONS WOMEN ASK WHEN THEY ARE PREGNANT

PAUL BWALYA

****

Blank page

****

Acknowledgement

To God my strength, I owe you everything

****

Blank page

****

Introduction

Pregnant women have a million questions they ask during pregnancy. They want to know why suddenly they are craving for soil, chalk and charcoal. They want to know why they have nausea; they want to know why they are vomiting. They want to know why they are having heartburn frequently. They want to know when they will feel the first kicks or heart beat of their unborn baby. Pregnancy is usually an exciting experience for women. It comes with a lot of anticipation and sometimes anxiety.

Pregnancy may also come with health disorders that if not prevented or attended to may pose a risk to both the mother and the unborn baby. Preventing and attending to these pregnancy associated health problems takes away anxiety and maximizes comfort through this experience.

In my decade long of practicing of midwifery at both community level and heath service delivery point in health facilities as a service provider, educator and clinical mentor, I have interacted with pregnant women from different walks of life. In this course of interaction, I have discussed with these women their several experiences while offering practical advice and answers to some questions and concerns they bring forward. This book looks at the 100 commonest questions women ask and answers to help a pregnant woman maximise their comfort during pregnancy

****

The first 1000 days of human life are considered most critical as the development that happens during this period determines the Physical and Psychosocial functioning of any human being for the rest of their lives.

The 1000 days are counted from the very day the baby is conceived. 270 days are in the womb, 365 days in the first year if life and 365 days in the second year of life.

This book also ensures that a pregnant woman takes her baby safely through the first 270 days in the womb while maximizing her comfort.

"Pregnancy is the only time when you can do nothing at all and still be productive." — Evan Esar

****

01 *HOW CAN I TELL THAT IAM PREGNANT?*

The commonest sign women notice and give them an intuition to suspect they are pregnant is when they have missed their monthly period. It is however so confusing especially for women with irregular periods. Menstruation is also affected by stress hormones and may be further delayed in an anxious and worrying woman. As much as a missed period is the first clue, you may look out for the following signs and symptoms.

Early Signs and symptoms

You may notice in a week or two after missing your periods that your breasts are tender and may be somehow itchy. On palpation, you may feel swollen lobes. This happens 4 weeks after conception

You may also experience an elevation in your temperature by 0.5 to 1 degrees Celsius. Progesterone hormone which is dominant in pregnancy is usually associated with rise in temperature whenever its levels in the body rise.

You may also notice that you are passing urine frequently than before as pregnancy hormones

****

overload the blood vessels by attracting extra water which is filtered off as urine in the kidneys.

Heart palpitations may also come in early as your heart pumps the increased blood volume faster.

However the surest way to confirm you're pregnant is a pregnancy test or an ultrasound scan.

"Everything grows rounder and wider and weirder, and I sit here in the middle of it all and wonder who in the world you will turn out to be." — Carrie Fisher

****

02   *IS IT POSSIBLE TO HAVE A FALSE PREGNANCY GROWING?*

It is very possible. A phantom or false pregnancy and may occur usually in women who so much desire to become pregnant. She may stop having monthly period and may present with some possible symptoms of pregnancy. The abdomen may actually be distended and breast may secrete some cloudy liquid.

This may occur because of the intense desire the woman may have to become pregnant. The part of the brain that is responsible for desiring and compassion sits next to the one the control pregnancy hormones which can be influenced to produce these pregnancy hormones and they affect the abdomen distending and are responsible for the symptoms of pregnancy we see.

However, the positive signs of pregnancy like the heart beat of the unborn baby which may only be picked by a midwife are absent. The pregnancy test is also likely to come out Negative as the chemical that the test kits pick are produced by the cells of a conceived baby.

****

Seeking specialized treatment from a psychologist or psychiatrist may be ideal in this case. And in instances where conception has delayed, seeking medical care from the specialised personel such a gynaecologist may help.

> "A ship under sail and a big-bellied woman are the handsomest two things that can be seen common."
> — Benjamin Franklin

03 IS IT POSSIBLE TO HAVE A FALSE NEGATIVE PREGNANCY TEST YET YOU'RE PREGNANT?

It is very possible to have a Negative test while you are pregnant. Pregnancy tests are designed to pick a hormone called Human Chorionic Gonadotrphin (HCG). This hormone is produced on the surface of the developing pre-baby cells. It takes about 2 weeks after conception before the hormone accumulates to levels that can be detected by your home test kit. If a test is done earlier than that, it may test negative due to low levels of HCG.

Repeating a pregnancy test a few days later may be advisable in this case.

"Before you were conceived I wanted you. Before you were born, I loved you. Before you were here an hour, I would die for you. This is the miracle of Mother's Love." — Maureen Hawkins

****

<h1>04 IS IT POSSIBLE TO HAVE A FALSE POSITIVE PREGNANCY TEST YET YOU'RE NOT PREGNANT?</h1>

Yes it is possible. Your test stripe may pick HCG which is circulating in blood but not really produced by the surface of the pre-baby cells in the womb. There are a couple of reasons why this may be the case.

A pregnancy test may be Positive in a case where woman has an ovarian cyst or Cancer with modified cell that may be producing a Chemical similar to HCG.

Certain medications may also be responsible for the false tests as they may contain elements that the test stripe may interpret as HCG from the growing baby. These include; Furosemide (a drug used in Blood Pressure control, Promethazine-used to control vomiting and diazepam also known as valium used to control anxiety and relaxing muscles.

You can also have a Positive pregnancy test after an abortion for a while as it may take some time to clear HCG hormone from your blood. It takes an average of 14 days to clear HCG from your blood after a miscarriage or the birth of the baby. It may

****

---

be longer than that or less depending on the levels of HCG hormone that accumulated.

> "A baby will make love stronger, days shorter, nights longer, bankroll smaller, home happier, clothes shabbier, the past forgotten and the future worth living for."— Unknown

05 WHY AM I HAVING HEARTBURN?

Heart burn is one of the commonest problem women have reported in early pregnancy. It is classified as a minor disorder in that it does not threaten the life of the woman. It however inversely affect the baby if the mothers nutrient intake if affected by the effects of heart burn.

Heartburn is a frequent complaint during pregnancy, reported by up to 72% of women during the last 3 months of pregnancy (Marrero et al 1992).

How does it come about?

For Pregnancy to reach term or delivery stage, it has to be sustained by relaxed muscles around the uterus and abdomen. There is a change in the hormone profile to ensure that this is achieved. A non-pregnant woman has dominantly high levels of oestrogen which mainly promote the growth of tissues and glands. However, if this was constantly the case in pregnancy, the uterine muscles will expel the baby before it reaches term or period of delivery. To counteract this effect, hormone progesterone relaxes the muscles in order to keep your baby until the point it will be able to survive outside the womb. However this hormone does not only relax the muscle of the uterus but even other muscles because it is transported in blood from the gland where it is produced. This includes muscles that prevent the contents of the stomach from moving backward. The stomach environment is acidic in nature because of the hydrochloric acid that is poured in there to aid digestion of the fats. The backflow of the acidic content leads to a burning sensation on the upper part of the stomach or around the lower sternum.

How can this be prevented?

Pregnancy is a period of adjustment for a woman in order to achieve comfort. You may be used to lying down flat in bed but this may worsen or predispose you to heartburn. Adopting a prop up position or sitting upright after meals with extra pillows on the head and back allows gravity to prevent backflow of acidic contents through the relaxed valve; a muscle that closes the stomach. Eating may be burdensome and uncomfortable in heartburn while keeping up with daily required nutrients at the same time hence taking frequent small meals to cover the daily intake may be helpful to avoid a small for age baby.

$$********$$

06 WHY AM I HAVING NAUSEA AND VOMITING?

About 85% of pregnant women experience nausea and 50% actual vomiting during pregnancy and a majority of them experience this between 6 weeks and 16 weeks into pregnancy (Jewell & Young 2003). It is believed that women carrying multiple babies may experience this more common than those carrying single ones.

Nausea and vomiting during pregnancy are often referred to as morning sickness despite women experiencing these symptoms throughout the day and/or night.

How does it come about?

Nausea and vomiting is highly associated with the rising of the hormone called Human Chorionic Gonadotrphin otherwise abbreviated as HCG which is produced from the surface of the fertilized ovum or egg. This hormone is intended to alert glands to produce enough progesterone to sustain your newly conceived baby before the placenta develops. However since it is also poured in blood, it affects other parts like the vomiting centre in the brain.

****

How can this be treated or prevented?

In mild cases, this is expected to go away on its own but you need to plan your meals in such a way that nausea and vomiting does not affect the intake of daily required fluids and nutrients. Food should be saved in environments free form other odours, well displayed and garnished. Small but frequent meals may be ideal.

In severe cases, a drug to treat vomiting usually one that counteracts dopamine in the brain such as Metoclopromide or Promethazine may be prescribed by your physician or midwife.

"A baby is something you carry inside you for nine months, in your arms for three years, and in your heart until the day you die." — Mary Mason

****

07 WHY AM I TAKING FOLIC ACID EVERYDAY?

Folic acid is one of the B-vitamins that are vital for the manufacture of White Blood Cells and Red Blood Cells in the human body. We normally get folic acid from green leafy vegetables and lentils such as beans and nuts. However supplementation in an event such as pregnancy is necessary.

Why is it that important in pregnancy?

Folic acid is especially important in pregnancy because it is not only needed for the manufacturing blood cells but also used in the manufacture of DNA which is used to manufacture proteins for the neural tube from which the brain and the spinal cord are formed. A deficiency in folic acid may therefore lead to deformities in the unborn baby related to the brain and spinal cord such as anencephaly where the baby is born without part of the brain and skull or spina bifida where the backbone that protects the spinal cord does not close completely.

****

08 *WHEN SHOULD I START TAKING FOLIC ACID?*

The defects associated with folic acid deficiency in the development of the unborn baby are incurred in the first few weeks of conception. The tube from which the brain and the spinal cord of your baby are developed is formed in the 3rd week after conceiving. A deficiency at this level may be catastrophic as it may lead to Neural Tube Defects such as anencephaly and spinal bifida.

It is recommended that women start Folic acid supplementation of 400mcg daily 4 weeks before becoming pregnant. However many women become pregnant without planning for that pregnancy. Women of child bearing age (15 - 49 years) are usually encouraged to add folic acid to their daily Vitamin supplementation so long they are in that age group.

"Pregnancy is getting company inside one's skin." — Maggie Scarf

****

09

SHOULD I TAKE FEROUS SULPHATE AS WELL SINCE AM TAKING FOLIC ACID?

Ferrous Sulphate is used in the treatment and prevention of anaemia. The Iron in ferrous sulphate is used to make healthy red blood cell. It is therefore important that a daily supplement of ferrous sulphate is taken as the demand is high in pregnancy.

World Health Organization recommends a daily supplementation of 60 mg elemental iron or an equivalent of 300mg Ferrous Sulphate in addition to 0.4 mg of Folic acid. Ferrous Sulphate is recommended for prevention of anaemia in pregnancy, infections, low birth weight and premature births.

A woman who has been found with low blood levels; below 10 g/dl is advised to increase the doses to 120 mg elemental iron until haemoglobin rise to above 10g/dl.

You need to understand that a woman with low blood level is also likely to bleed while give birth and this is one of the leading causes of maternal deaths.

****

10 WHY AM I CRAVING FOR SOIL AND CHARCOAL?

Some pregnant women usually experience weird and strange craving for non food substances such as soil, ashes, charcoal and many weird substance. This is a condition we call *Pica.* Pica is originally a Latin word for a bird known as a **Magpie.** It is believed that a Magpie can eat almost anything.

What causes Pica

Pica is associated with the deficiency from of Iron which usually drops in pregnancy in an event where supplementation is not done. The consequences may be bad for women who give in to this craving and opt to be eating soil. Soil may contain eggs for worms and may lead to an infestation. This may worsen the situation as blood sucking worms may cause anaemia and further deficiency of iron.

How can this be prevented?

Ferrous Sulphate supplementation which contains iron may be used for both prevention and treatment of anaemia.

****

11 WHY AM I FREQUENTLY PASSING URINE?

Many pregnant women experience frequency in passing urine especially in the first 12 weeks of pregnancy and the last 4 weeks before delivery. This may be inconveniencing but works somehow to your advantage. Frequency in passing urine helps to clean the lower passages and prevent infections in both the urine passes and lower birth canal.

How does it come about?

The pregnancy hormones progesterone and Human Chorionic Gonadotrophin attract a lot of water in the blood stream that pass through the kidney. This makes it possible for the body to filter off more urine from the blood. Secondly; the pregnant uterus is positioned in the same cavity with the bladder hence it can't get to full capacity because of limited space. This makes it to be emptying more frequently.

Can it be prevented?

No, this comes about naturally and will reduce at around 12 weeks in pregnancy as the pregnant

$$********$$

womb will move out of the pelvic cavity into the abdomen around this time.

> "Pregnancy is a process that invites you to surrender to the unseen force behind all life." — Judy Ford

$$********$$

<table>
<tr><td>

12

</td><td>

WHY IS MY FACE DARKENNING? IT FEELS SO THICK LIKE AM PUTTING ON A MASK?

</td></tr>
</table>

As much exciting pregnancy can be, women experience a lot of changes in the bodies and some of them may be less comfortable but for a short period of time. Hyper pigmentation of the skin during pregnancy is very common, occurring in up to 90% of pregnant women. Hyper pigmentation results in a darkening of areas that are already pigmented. It is usually more noticeable in women with dark complexions (Muallem & Rubeiz 2006)

Hormones may cause brown parches on your face, and body. This condition is known as ***Chloasma*** while others refer to this as The ***Mask of pregnancy.***

Can this be treated?

The hormones responsible for this are still needed at high levels in the body in order to sustain the pregnancy. However, avoiding excessive exposure to the sun may help to stop the condition from worsening. You may need a hat during sunny day.

****

13   *WHY AM I HAVING EXCESS STRETCH MARKS?*

Many pregnant women develop stretch marks during pregnancy. It is actually estimated that 8 in 10 pregnant women have stretch marks. They appear lighter than your skin on your tummy and thighs.

How do they come about?

There is rapid growth of tissues in pregnancy due to enlargement and multiplication of body cells. This is aided by the rising levels of pregnancy hormones.

"Think of stretch marks as pregnancy service stripes." – Joyce Armo

14 HOW DO I GET RID OF STRETCH MARKS?

Once your baby is born, the marks may gradually fade away and become less noticeable. In a case where you are experience some itching that may come with the stretching. Some oils may be useful.

There is however no treatment for the stretch marks and even after delivery there will still be some that will remain. Some tissues will get back to normal as early as six weeks after birth of the baby. Exercising mildly like taking walks may actually expedite this process and aid the body to come back to near normal.

> "Your pregnant elephant ankles will return to normal. Just hang in there." — Adriel Booker

$$\text{\Large ********}$$

15

WHY AM I HAVING ACNE (PIMPLES)?

A good number of women may have acne during pregnancy. It usually occurs early in pregnancy especially in the first 3 to 6 months in pregnancy. Many pregnant women attempt to clear this as soon as possible. Some of the measures you may take may actually just worsen the situation.

How does it come about?

During pregnancy, there is a surge of hormones such Human Chorionic Gonadotrophin (HCG) and Progesterone among others. These hormones enable the glands to in your skin including those of your face which produce oil. The increased oil being produced clog up the pores which then become invasion by bacteria and inflammation.

How to prevent it?

Many may be tempted to do facial scrubbing and steaming but that may just stimulate the glands to even produce more oil. Many oral Medications should also be avoided especially in early pregnancy. Acne clears out when the hormone levels begin to go down. Towards the end of pregnancy both HCG and progesterone begin to down. A mild soap with lukewarm water may be Ideal. Increased fluid intake to promote the flow in those moths is recommended.

"We can't understand when we're pregnant, or when our siblings are expecting, how profound it is to have a shared history with a younger generation: blood, genes, humor. It means we were actually here, on Earth, for a time—like the Egyptians with their pyramids, only with children." — Anne Lamott

16 WHY AM I HAVING CONSTIPATION?

Constipation is the condition in which a person has difficulties in eliminating solid waste from the body.

How does this happen?

Once food is ingested, it is propelled down by the body through a process called peristalsis. This is the contraction and relaxation muscles around the food passages. During pregnancy, the hormone progesterone relaxes muscles including those around the intestines which make the flow to be sluggish. This is was leads to constipation. Although it initially gives some form of advantage to the pregnant woman as maximum nutrients are absorbed from the food, it may lead to constipation which is a health problem.

How can this be prevented?

Dietary modifications play a very important role in ensuring that constipation and other health problems are avoided. A diet rich in fibre such as fruits, vegetables, cereals and lentils help in preventing constipation. Increasing of fluid intake also helps in the prevention of constipation. A pregnant woman should take at least 8 glasses of water every day. Mild exercises also helps to keep the muscles active hence helps in preventing constipation. She can take walks or swim regularly.

"Sometimes the smallest things take up the most room in your heart." — A.A. Milne

****

17   *WHY AM I SPOTTING (BLEEDING)? IS THAT NORMAL?*

A woman should not bleed while she is pregnant. Bleeding in pregnancy can be a bad sign. It may indicate an impending miscarriage. However, very little drops may be visible approximately 10 days after conception. This is normal and happens the time the fertilized egg is implanting or nesting in the uterus tissue.

How does it happen?

Fertilization of the egg occurs in the fallopian tube where the sperms meet the released ovum/egg. There after rapid multiplication of the fertilized egg occurs into what may look like a mulberry. It then embarks on a 10 days journey to the uterus where the unborn baby is sheltered. When the tiny mulberry like baby reaches the uterus it usually sticks to the upper wall of the uterus. It then digests the lining of the uterus which is richly supplied with blood vessels in order to create a nest for itself. This process is what leads to spotting. However the blood is very minimal as compared to when a woman is having a monthly period. There may be slight lower abdominal cramps less painful than what a woman may experience when having a monthly period.

In an event of bleeding

If it happens that bleeding occurs outside the 10 days period after conception and in larger quantities, it may be an impending miscarriage and precautions should be taken to preserve the pregnancy. The woman should immediately visit a Midwife or a doctor who determines the outcome after examination has been done. Rest may be recommendation in this case.

"When I was pregnant, I was so huge and people on the bus would get up for me. That made me feel so precious and valued and valuable. I try to treat everyone like they're pregnant." — Mariska Hargitay

****

18   *WHEN SHOULD MY BABY IN THE WOMB START KICKING*

The kicking baby in the womb may be used as a good assurance that the baby is doing fine. It is usually a joyful moment to feel the first kick and it just freak women out.

When does it happen?

Doctors and Midwives use the term *'quickening'* to refer to the very first kick your baby makes in the womb. The best time to look out for it usually, depends on whether you had a baby before of not. For women who are pregnant for the first time it take a little bit longer that the one who had a baby before. Women who have had babies before usually start feeling the baby kicking at 16 weeks after conception while those pregnant for the first time usually at 20 weeks after conception.

> "No matter how bad my day's been, it takes one little kick to make everything feel alright." – *Author Unknown*

19 *HOW OFTEN SHOULD THE BABY KICK?*

The kicking in the womb is not only used to confirm that the woman is indeed pregnant but may also indicate how well the baby may be. The baby must kick at least 10 to 12 times in a single. Too many kicks or very little may indicate the baby is receiving too little oxygen and is in distress.

Many conditions may cause the baby to receive low oxygen. These may include the mother having conditions which may reduce oxygen carrying capacity such as anaemia or smoking.

If you suspect your baby is not kicking much or is kicking too much. It's time to visit your midwife of doctor.

A midwife at your health service facility may check the heart beat of you baby and the number, frequency and regularity of the beat may help determine how well your baby may be doing.

****

20 WHY AM I LOOKING A LITTLE BIT PALE?

A lot of changes happen in almost all the systems in your body during pregnancy. These changes also happen in the blood concentrations. There is an initial increase in the amount of blood during pregnancy but in an imbalanced manner.

The liquid component increase more than the solid component in the first three to six months in pregnancy. This increase in the fluid component cause dilution of blood making the pregnant woman skin appears pale. It is estimated that the fluid component rise by 50% while the solid component only rise by 20%. The solid component then keeps on increasing in the 4th to the 9th month.

It should be noted however that if the concentration of the blood does not improve, it may affect the delivery of oxygen to the baby and consequently the growth and wellbeing of the baby. World Health Organization recommends that a pregnant woman should have Haemoglobin concentration of at least 10 g/dl. Pregnant women who have low haemoglobin are also likely to bleed much before, during and after delivery as platelets which are the

****

clotting agents are part of the solid component of blood.

> "Rigid plans work best if you're building a skyscraper; with something as mysteriously human as giving birth, it's best, both literally and figuratively, to keep your knees bent." — Mark Sloan

****

21   *WHY AM I HAVING WHITE SECRETIONS ON THE PRIVATE PART NOW?*

A good number of pregnant women I have attended to during my antenatal clinics have reported excess white discharge from the vagina during pregnancy. It is a source of worry to many in pregnancy and cause of stress.

It should however be noted that it is quite normal to have excess discharge during pregnancy. It should also be noted that this usually white discharge should be non-offensive and non-irritating.

The increase in the white discharge commonly referred to as Leucorrhoea is highly associated with increase in hormones such as progesterone during pregnancy. The pregnant woman may just need to wash her private part with clean water only. NO MEDICATED soap. Vaginal douching and use of tampons should also be avoided.

However, if the increase in discharge is associated with itching, soreness, offensive smell, or pain when passing urine, the underlying cause should be determined (NICE 2008).

Bacterial, fungal and viral infections may also affect the pregnant woman. These may include vaginal candidiasis and bacterial vaginosis which may also present with a white discharge but comes with itching and soreness, pain on passing urine and may be foul smelling. In this case seeking treatment from a health facility where laboratory investigation may be done to find the cause and appropriate treatment.

. "A good way to prepare yourself for parenthood is to talk to rocks because they have similar listening habits." — Rodney Lacroix

****

22 WHY AM I HAVING SWOLLEN VEINS AT THE BACK OF MY LEGS?

You may experience, swollen veins behind your legs as it may be the case with many other pregnant women especially from month 5 or 6 till after delivery. They may look twisted like a tree.

How do they come about?

The hormone progesterone softens the walls of the blood vessels. The blood vessels mainly affected are the veins because they carry blood back to the heart uphill against gravity. The relaxed blood vessels fail to clear up the blood which leads to accumulation. This is worsened by additional pressure that the growing pregnancy puts on the major veins at the back of the womb especially if a pregnant woman lies on her back.

How can I prevent them?

Engaging in activities that will promote blood circulation is key to prevention; these may include, mild exercises such as daily walk, elevating the foot end when lying down with a pillow or two, putting on compression stockings may also help.

****

However, as soon as you deliver and the hormone levels begin to drop in a week or two, your legs goes back to normal.

> "My body has given me the greatest gift of my life." — Hilary Duff

****

23 WHY DO I NEED TO WIDEN UP TO BALANCE? MY STEP HAS CHANGED

Many ligaments in the body including those around the spinal cord tend to loosen up during pregnancy. This is believed to be brought about by a change in the hormone profile of a pregnant woman. A hormone called relaxin and progesterone are largely thought to be responsible for this and usually change the pregnant woman's posture and is the main causes of back and pelvic pain during pregnancy.

Posture is altered as the pregnancy grows because the curvature of the lower spine becomes exaggerated to accommodate the ever increasing weight of the pregnant womb. The Centre of gravity which sits directly above the middle of the base of a human being at this point shift in a pregnant. This may require a pregnant woman to widen up their base balance and this usually happens subconsciously. In trying to find relief for the pain and balance the extra weight of the growing baby a pregnant woman may subconsciously adopt a unique walking style known as a **'wadding gait'**

****

Less strenuous and pregnant-specific exercises as well as physiotherapy have shown to reduce back or pelvic pain, whilst some women reported pain relief by using pillows to support their stomachs when lying down. Back strain may be reduced by women turning onto their sides when sitting up and as they swing their legs down when they get up off a couch or bed.

> . "Life is tough enough without having someone kick you from the inside." Rita Rudner

24 WHY AM I FEELING LIKE I HAVE PINS IN MY HANDS

Blood vessels are equally not an exemption to the relaxing effects of pregnancy hormones that rise in the blood during pregnancy. Blood vessels, especially the veins become relaxed and this reduces the speed of blood returning back to the heart. This sluggish movement gives an advantage to the pregnant womans body as maximum amount of absorbed nutrient are used up by the body cells. Fluids that carry these nutrients move from blood vessels in the tissues and eventually body cells. This fluid which keeps on accumulating in very small quantities may eventually cause swelling and pain in the hands. This affects the nerves in the hands and the pregnant woman may feel like pins in the hands.

In order to reduce this and promote comfort, wrist splints as well as mild non steroid analgesia may be used. Mild hand exercises such as a small cotton or rubber ball. A physiotherapist may provide more guidance in severe cases.

****

25   *CAN I TAKE STILL TAKE ALCOHOL?*

As much as some may advise you that some small amount of alcohol may still be consumed during pregnancy. It may be dangerous as a onetime exposure may bring effects that may affect the baby for a life time. People breakdown alcohol molecules different and the same amount considered small in one person may be disastrous in another one.

How does it affect the baby?

Alcohol is able to cross barriers and go into the baby's blood circulation. It then in turn brings about what is called Foetal Alcohol Syndrome. This affect mental and intellectual and cognitive development of the unborn baby and the damage incurred may be permanent. This is observed in someone's childhood. Sign and symptoms may include; speech and language difficulties, low birth weight, mental illness, small head and brain and behavioural disorders.

Excessive alcohol intake is potentially lethal, affecting virtually every organ and system in the body, including the liver, gastrointestinal tract, and

****

cardiovascular and neurological systems. It affects nutrition by suppressing the appetite and by altering the metabolism, mobilization and storage of nutrients (Wardlow 2000).

Excessive or chronic alcohol abuse is associated with several vitamin and mineral deficiencies, including folic acid, vitamin B, magnesium and iron all of them much needed in the period of organ formation and development in the womb.

Learning difficulties, loss of memory and other mental problems are associated with infants born to parents who have abused alcohol (Chang et al 1998).

Women's tolerance of alcohol is lower than that of men because of differences in body size, absorption and metabolism. They have a higher proportion of fat to water; therefore alcohol becomes more concentrated in body fluids and damaging effects such as gastritis, pancreatitis, peptic ulcers and malnutrition are more likely to develop. Drinking alcohol during pregnancy is both affect formation of the baby's body parts and maybe poisonous to the baby in the womb

****

26   *CAN I STILL TAKE ICECREAM WHILE IAM PREGNANT?*

A lot of pregnant women have different cravings of food and sometimes weird non-food substances. Ice cubes and Ice cream is one such common stuff women crave for during pregnancy. It is however still safe to take ice creams if it is taken once in a while considering it is made from pasteurized milk with no caffeine added and shouldn't be taken daily during this period.

Too much of it however may lead to some problems and should be taken with much consideration. The sugar in the ice cream may predispose the woman to pregnancy related diabetes and its associated complications including a big baby which may lead to a difficulty delivery as well.

There is also a risk of putting on too much weight which is undesirable in pregnancy. A weight addition of more than 500g per week in the 4th month to the 9th Month may pose a risk including raised blood Pressure and convulsions.

27 CAN I TAKE AN ENERGY DRINK WHILE AM TILL PREGNANT.

Energy drinks usually contain high levels of sugar, caffeine and preservatives and they are usually carbonated. All of these are not encouraged during pregnancy. High sugar may predispose a pregnant woman to gaining excess weight and pregnancy related diabetes as well as hypertension.

Caffeine clearance in pregnancy is reduced; hence even amounts that may be considered normal in a non-pregnant person may affect a pregnant woman.

It has also been largely associated with small babies for their age, still births and preterm births.

> "It is the most powerful creation to have life growing inside of you..." — Beyoncé

28. CAN I STILL TAKE CHOCOLATE IN PREGNANCY?

Chocolate can be consumed in moderation during pregnancy as well. Some studies conducted have actually indicated that chocolate in moderation during pregnancy may reduce the risk of hypertension associated with pregnancy.

However, consuming large amounts of chocolate may also affect pregnancy. Chocolate like coffee and tea also contains considerable amount of caffeine which may affect pregnancy. In addition to this, it also contains sugar that may lead to excess weight during pregnancy and this is undesirable as it is associated with many complications

"Making the decision to have a baby is momentous. It is to decide forever to have your heart go walking around outside your body." –

****

29 CAN I STILL TAKE COFFEE IN PREGNANCY?

Coffee is one of the widely consumed beverages across the globe. The craving for coffee may be irresistible sometime, but how safe is coffee during pregnancy?

According to the World health Organization, caffeine is a stimulant found in tea, coffee, soft drinks, chocolate, kola nuts, energy drinks and some over the counter medications.

Coffee is one of the most common sources of high caffeine intake. During pregnancy, caffeine clearance from the mother's blood slows down significantly. Results from some observational studies suggest that excess intake of caffeine may be associated with growth restriction of the unborn baby, reduced birth weight, premature labour and still births (WHO 2016)

It is recommended that pregnant women with high daily caffeine intake lower their daily caffeine intake during pregnancy to reduce the risk of pregnancy loss and low birth weight babies

****

30   *CAN I STILL CONTINUE SMOKING WHILE AM PREGNANT?*

Smoking is one of the addictive habits that may be difficult to pause. However, if you are a smoker and you become pregnant you need to look at these recommendations again.

Centre for Disease Control and Prevention (CDC) revealed that; Women who smoke have more difficulty becoming pregnant and have a higher risk of never becoming pregnant.

Smoking during pregnancy can harm the unborn baby, particularly in the lung and brain and some studies suggests a link between maternal smoking and cleft lip.

Studies also suggest a relationship between tobacco and miscarriage. Carbon monoxide in tobacco smoke can keep the developing baby from getting enough oxygen. Tobacco smoke also contains other chemicals that can harm unborn babies. One in every five babies born to mothers who smoke during pregnancy has low birth weight

****

31 HOW MUCH FLUIDS SHOULD I TAKE DAILY NOW THAT I AM PREGNANT?

Fluid intake is very important during pregnancy as it helps to keep the woman hydrated and strong.

It is recommended that a pregnant woman takes at least 8 to 12 glasses of water every day.

Foods with plenty of fluids like water melons, cucumbers and pineapples are encouraged during this period.

Smoothies and raw fruits are may help to rehydrate the mother.

> "What good mothers and fathers instinctively feel like doing for their babies is usually best after all." –
>
> *Benjamin Spock*

****

32   WHY SHOULD I INCREASE FLUID INTAKE?

Apart from ensuring rehydration is maximized during pregnancy; it is worth noting that an increase in fluid intake helps in the formation of amniotic fluid which cushions and protect the unborn baby in an event of shock.

Extra fluids help in the removal of excess waste from blood through the kidneys. It also helps to prevent infections in the urinary tract, the bladder and the kidneys as the urine flashes these systems. It also helps to prevent crystal formation in the relaxed urinary system.

The movement of the contents of the intestines are reduced to allow maximum absorption of nutrients. This however predisposes a pregnant woman to constipation. An increase in water and fluid intake helps to prevent this as stool is softened.

****

33 *CAN I STILL TAKE SPICES WHILE AM PREGNANT*

Many pregnant women about 72% experience heart burn which is brought about stomach contents flowing back through the relaxed sphincter muscles of the upper part of the stomach which controls food moving back in the oesophagus.

Spicy foods may add much discomfort if this happened as they will increase heart burn.

Women with heart burn are not encouraged to take spices, coffee or carbonated drinks for this reason.

> "To be pregnant is to be vitally alive, thoroughly woman, and distressingly inhabited. Soul and spirit are stretched – along with body – making pregnancy a time of transition, growth, and profound beginnings."– *Anne*

34 — HOW MANY HOURS SHOULD I SLEEP PER DAY?

Any activity in pregnancy that increases the uptake of energy depreciates the much needed oxygen for both the mother and the baby. The primary purpose is to conserve energy and allow more oxygen to the baby so that the growth can be optimized.

Rest is therefore important in pregnancy to reduce the metabolic rate and conserve energy. A pregnant woman should sleep for a minimum of 8 hours day but sleeping more than 10 hours may make her inactive and predispose her to many other problems including a further drop in the immune system and pregnancy disorder like swollen veins on the back of the legs much associated with inactivity.

Low oxygen levels crossing to the baby may lead to condition unborn babies suffers from in low oxygen environment called *foetal distress.* This may even result in the death of the baby in the womb.

****

35   *WHICH POSITION IS MORE COMFORTABLE TO SLEEP IN WHEN YOU'RE PREGNANT?*

With the fatigue that pregnancy may come with and the need to conserve more energy in pregnancy, adopting the most comfortable position for you helps you to maximize your rest.

As a midwife I always start training my clients from the earliest possible time to adopt the ideal position even before the pregnancy grows.

Sleeping on the left side has been widely seen not only to promote comfort since it relieves pressure of an average 1.5 kg liver off the major blood vessel hence promoting circulation.

Promoting blood circulation in turn prevents many other problems in pregnancy such as sluggish movement of blood in veins; varicose veins and swelling of feet.

Sleeping on the back may also affect the health of your unborn baby. The weight of your unborn baby, the womb and the fluid around the baby weighs over 7 kg together and may exert pressure on the blood vessel that deliver oxygen to your unborn baby in the womb.

****

> "Babies are bits of star-dust blown from the hand of God. Lucky is the woman who knows the pangs of birth for she has held a star." – *Larry Barretto*

****

36 — *DO I NEED TO CONTINUE WITH MY ROUTINE EXERCISES NOW THAT I AM PREGNANT?*

As much as energy conservation is cardinal in pregnancy, inactivity may bring its own problems in pregnancy. Exercises have benefits that may prevent a lot of problems. M

What type of exercises can I do them?

Less strenuous exercises can be done in pregnancy and these include swimming which is both less strenuous to the woman and cannot pose risk of injury to the baby. A pregnant woman can also take walks to keep the tone of her muscles strong and also helps to strengthen the immune system.

> "I'm never as happy as when I'm pregnant. I literally would have 10 babies if I could!"
> – *Tori Spelling*

37 — *CAN I STILL PUT ON HIGH HEELS WHILE AM PREGNANT?*

Putting on high heels during pregnancy not only put the baby at risk in case of a slip and fall but also predisposes the pregnant woman to problems that may come with pregnancy.

During pregnancy, the centre of gravity of a woman shift downwards and forward. This makes her to lose balance somehow. Putting on heels further makes her unstable and she risk falling.

Secondly, women experience what is called *lordosis* where the lower backbone bends forward. This may come with some backache in women. This condition is made much worse with a woman who puts on heals.

****

38 *WHY DO I FEEL SO EXHAUSTED?*

Fatigue or exhaustion are very much common and affect almost every pregnant woman especially in the first 3 months of pregnancy. It is actually one of the earliest symptoms women experience. Some experience this as early as a week after conception of the baby.

Fatigue usually comes about as a result of increased energy demand in the formation of the baby in the womb. This requires extra nutrients, oxygen supply and other raw materials.

Taking at least one extra hour of rest during the day is recommended for a pregnant woman and an extra hour of sleep in the night in order to conserve this much needed energy.

Eating small frequent meals will constantly provide the body with the energy needs.

Co-existing condition such as anaemia or asthma that may lead to the reduction the blood carrying capacity of oxygen may worsen fatigue. It recommended that anaemia is prevented or treated during pregnancy.

****

39 WHY DO I HAVE THIS BACKACHE?

Many factors contribute to the pain in the back when a woman is pregnant. Slightly more than half of the pregnant women experience back especially after four months from conception.

Firstly pregnancy hormones soften the discs and ligaments that hold the bones of the backbone in their place. The lower part of the backbone then begins to bend forward and down from the weight of both the trunk and the growing womb. This usually put a strain on the lower backbone and cause pain. There is strong evidence to suggest that about 20% of pregnant women experience this pain (Vleeming et al 2008).

This pain may occur in the lower back, hips and groins, and it is commonly triggered by standing on one leg while climbing stairs, dressing, getting in and out of the bath or turning in bed (ACPWH 2007a).

This pain is mainly managed by physiotherapy and mild exercises such as swiming, a pelvic belt for

****

---

short periods and some analgesia may be used Current

Back and pelvic pain are common in pregnancy, with up to 76% of women reporting back pain at some point during their pregnancy (Kristiansson et al 1996).

"Babies are always more trouble than you thought—and more wonderful." — Charles Osgood

.

40 IS IT OKAY TO LIE ON MY BACK WHILE PREGNANT?

Women need to constantly adjust during pregnancy especially as the pregnancy grows. Lying on the back is not encouraged in pregnancy except during the examination of the abdomen and she not encouraged to be in that position for a long time. It affects both the baby and the mother. The weight acquired during pregnancy may especially that of the unborn baby, the pregnant uterus and the amniotic fluid may apply pressure on the major blood vessels including those that supply oxygenated blood to the baby. This may negatively affect the wellbeing of the baby.

The woman may also be affected by a condition called supine hypotension where blood pressure drops because of this position and perfusion of oxygen to vital organs like the brain is reduced as well and she may feel the dizziness.

I usually train my clients to first turn on the side then drop their legs before getting off the couch from the very first session to ensure this sink down the mind.

41   *IS OKAY TO TAKE HOT SHOWER?*

Long hot showers may be something you frequently enjoy to take in your routine lifestyle but pregnancy comes with adaptations to ensure that you and your unborn baby navigate safely through this journey.

Hot showers may lead to the heating up of the body above 38 degrees Celsius and this temperature is not recommended in a pregnant woman especially in the first months in pregnancy. Over heating the body may lead to some brain and spinal cord malformations in the unborn baby. It may also lead to dehydration as well.

It is recommended that a pregnant woman takes a warm shower and not a long hot shower.

> "Now my belly is as noble as my heart." — Gabriela Mistral

****

42   *IAM VOMITING EXCESSIVELY, AM I EXPECTING TWINS?*

Nausea and vomiting is common especially early in pregnancy. Pregnant women lose some fluids and electrolytes if this continues for a long time. Food intake may also be reduced and this may lead to hypoglycaemia. Small frequent meals are therefore advised with plenty of fluids.

Nausea and vomiting has been observed to be more common in women who lack vitamin B6, magnesium and Zinc.

Some studies suggest that due to the large placenta area taken by the twins, more hormones are likely to be produced and a woman carrying twins may experience much nausea and vomiting as compared to the one carrying a single baby.

****

43 MY FEET ARE SWOLLEN, AM I EXPECTING TWINS?

So many superstitions are linked to pregnancy and swelling of the feet is one of them. Some people in some cultures believe that when a woman has swollen feet she could be carrying twins.

Swollen feet in pregnancy may be a sign of something that needs further investigations. Because of the dilution of blood that happens this may be however be expected.

Swelling of feet may come because of the relaxed veins and resultant slowed return of blood back to the heart. This allows fluids to move out of the veins into the tissues.

A woman with anaemia or hypertension linked to pregnancy can present with swollen feet. And sometimes it just happens that when there is pressure in the veins fluids returns in the tissues even without blood pressure rising or having anaemia.

****

44 AM I SUPPOSED TO TAKE ANY MEDICATION WHEN AM SICK WHILE

Medication during pregnancy should be approached with caution. Before a pregnant woman thinks about medication for any ailment the benefits and the risks of taking such medication should first be reviewed.

From day 0–14 days after conception, a period before the conceived baby is nested in the womb, some medication may be tolerated though those with long term effects will still affect the baby at that early age and even result in the death of the baby.

It has been observed that many medications taken at 2 weeks may actually cause you to abort the baby you have just conceived.

After two weeks or 18 days to 55 days, many parts of your unborn baby begin to form. This is the period when pregnancy is vulnerable to several drugs and some medications at this stage will cause malformations in your unborn baby. Some medications or drugs that are administered later after this stage of pregnancy including alcohol,

****

cocaine, insulin, furosemide, and antithyroid agents may damage the newly formed organs before they even mature.

It is therefore recommended that a pregnant woman should never take any medication that has not been prescribed by a physician or a midwife

> "If I had my life to live over, instead of wishing away nine months of pregnancy, I'd have cherished every moment and realised that the wonderment growing inside me was the only chance in life to assist God in a miracle." – ***Erma Bombeck***

****

45   IS IT POSSIBLE TO TELL MY BABY IS DOING FINE DURING PREGNANCY?

Just the way we check your Blood pressure and heart rate at the prenatal clinic, we also check the vital signs of your unborn babies to determine how fine they are doing. Some of the things we look out for include the heart rate and we are able to tell that a particular deviation from the normal may indicate for instance low oxygenation in your unborn baby causing distress.

We also check and teach pregnant women to ensure they pay attention to how frequent the baby is kicking in the womb because as a midwife I always ask for this information to help me determine how well your baby is doing.

A baby that is receiving good nutrients and oxygen should kick at least 10 to 12 times in 12 hours. Too much of that or too few may indicate distress.

In a situation where a pregnant woman expresses concern of feeling few baby kicks or movements, a kick Chart may be used to ensure the correct assessment is done. The cessation of the kicks may indicate the death of the unborn baby in the womb

****

46 WHAT DRUGS SHOULD I AVOID IN PREGNANCY?

As a midwife I always say a pregnant woman should avoid every drug as long as it has not been prescribed by the physician or a midwife. Drugs that may normally be taken by everyone including alcohol, cocaine, insulin, Furosemide, aspirin, and antithyroid agents may have devastating effects on pregnancy.

Drugs in pregnancy are prescribed based on assessment of risks and benefits and that should only be done by a midwife or physician at your health centre.

> "You do a lot of growing up when you're pregnant. It's suddenly like, 'Yikes. Here it is, folks. Playtime is over.'" — Connie Fioretto

****

47

I HAVE CONCEIVED TOO EARLY, SHOULD I CONTINUE BREASTFEEDING THE OTHER CHILD?

It is very safe to breast feed while you're pregnant. Neither the pregnant woman nor the pregnancy is harmed in any way.

Breastfeeding is an important practice from the very first hour the baby is born. All the nutrients the baby needs in the first 6 months of life including water and the first immunity from diseases that the baby receives is passed to them through breast milk.

At the age 6 months other foods in form of purees and porridge may be introduced to complement to the energy needs that the baby needs at this age. Breast milk however still remains a very important source of nutrients until when the baby completes a critical 1000 days from conceptions at the age of 2 years.

Stopping breast feeding at any point in this period without a sustainable replacement nutrients found in breast milk may be catastrophic.

48 IS IT OKAY TO USE INSECTICISIDE WHILE AM PREGNANT?

Fumigating a house that where an occupant is pregnant should highly be reconsidered especially in the first 3 months of pregnancy. Once inhaled some chemicals that are used as insecticides may have an effect in the formation of the baby parts especially the spinal cord and the brain.

In mosquito infested areas, the pregnant woman still needs protections against mosquito bites which transmit malaria. A long lasting insecticide treated net is recommended as opposed to the use of insecticide sprays in a room where the pregnant woman is sleeping.

****

49 WHEN AM I SUPPOSED TO STOP MAKING LOVE NOW THAT AM EXPECTING?

Sex during pregnancy has been shrouded in myths and misconceptions in many cultures and traditions across the globe. In the traditional British antenatal care, it was advised that a couple abstain although without any evidence to substantiate this stance.

During pregnancy, many couples are fearful of continuing their sexual relationship. They may feel that they may somehow provoke miscarriage, premature labour or damage the fetus; some men have expressed fear of breaking the 'bag of waters' (Kitzinger 1985).

In the Zambia tradition, sex is only encouraged in early pregnancy. It is believed that semen deposited in late pregnancy during sexual intercourse sticks to the baby's skin and is very difficult to clear off.

Sex has however no effect on pregnancy and can be performed by couple so the woman is comfortable

and not straining. Sex positions that are comfortable may be explored to avoid stress.

****

50   *DOES SEMEN AFFECT THE UNBORN CHILD IN ANYWAY?*

Semen does not affect your unborn baby in any way. Contrary to myths and misconception that shroud sex in pregnancy, Sex is safe during pregnancy.

Firstly you need to understand that there is no contact between semen and your unborn baby. The unborn baby is safely protected in a bag of waters that is surrounded by several layers which acts as a barrier to the outside environment.

In addition to these barriers, the uterus is closed by a plug of mucus during pregnancy and this is only released when a woman goes in labour.

"When you moved, I felt squeezed with a wild infatuation and protectiveness. We are one. Nothing, not even death, can change that."– Suzanne Finnamore

****

51 CAN I STILL TAKE CARBONATED DRINKS NOW THAT IAM PREGNANT?

Carbonate drinks are not encouraged during pregnancy because of their content in relation to the physical changes that the woman undergoes during the period of pregnancy.

Pregnant women are likely to suffer from heart burn because of the effect of hormones on muscles closing the stomach. Carbonated drinks are likely to trigger or aggravate this effect. Some may contain caffeine which is associated with restricted growth of the baby in the uterus.

Many artificial sweeteners and colorants that are used in these drinks may contain chemicals that are not recommended in pregnancy. They may be small amounts but absorption during pregnancy is enhanced and these same amounts may be harmful.

Pure juices and well pasteurized milk are smoothies may be taken. Fresh fruits in addition may also be recommended.

****

52

The weight of your unborn baby can be estimated and compared to the age of your unborn baby counting from conception. A physician or a midwife may then help you to determine whether the weight is appropriate for the age.

Foetal weight estimation can be made by using measurements obtained during ultrasound assessment.

Knowing the estimated weight of your unborn baby through an ultrasound scan may help you seek appropriate advice and care from the specialised health personnel.

Where a premature birth is eminent, this information may help you to understand why some interventions may be recommended as the weight of your unborn baby guides the process.

****

53

CAN I TAKE WATER TREATED WITH CHLORINE WHILE AM STILL PREGNANT?

Chlorine is one of the commonest chemical used for water purification. Pregnant women have raised concern on the safety of this water purification agent.

Its safety can still not totally be guaranteed especially in the first 3 months of pregnancy. Some studies have associated unborn babies who are small for their age to use of chlorine in pregnancy.

It is recommended that the amount of chlorine in drinking water should not exceed 0.05% and testing from the water source should be done to ensure the amount is within acceptable levels.

> "Life is always a rich and steady time when you are waiting for something to happen or to hatch."– *E.B. White,Charlotte's*

****

54 *I HAVE HIV; WILL I INFECT MY UNBORN BABY?*

HIV is transmitted largely through sexual intercourse, infected piercing instruments like needles and it can be transmitted from the mother to a child during pregnancy, child birth or breastfeeding if no intervention is taken.

If interventions are started in pregnancy by initiating a pregnant woman on antiretro viral treatment, it eliminates the chance of infecting the child in the womb.

Antiretroviral treatment reduces the virus amount in the body to a level where it cannot be transmitted to the baby in the womb or during child birth or breastfeeding. This usually happens as long as the mother is adhering to the treatment.

The blood of the unborn baby is does not mix in normal circumstances as the placenta creates a selective barrier. The risk is usually higher during child birth and there is need to ensure that the amounts of viruses in the body are reduced to safer levels.

****

The baby born from a mother with HIV is also given antiretro viral treatment as post exposure treatment to ensure that every chance is eliminated

> "There is a sanctity involved with bringing a child into this world, it is better than bombing one out of it. – *James Baldwin*

55   *I TESTED POSITIVE FOR SYPHILI; WILL IT AFFECT MY UNBORN BABY?*

Syphilis is one of the diseases that are screened by the midwives or clinicians during antenatal care clinics. The objective is to detect these diseases early and treat them.

During the primary or secondary stage of syphilis, transmission to the unborn baby will inevitably occur at any stage of pregnancy. Complications include miscarriage, stillbirth, premature delivery, and congenital syphilis, and 50% of babies born to these infected women will die within 4 weeks (Heffner & Schust 2006).

Organism that cause syphilis can also damage the placenta barrier and provide entry of other bacteria and viruses like HIV

It is therefore, recommended that you get treatment from your nearest health facility as soon as possible.

Once it is treated early no complications are usually noted and babies are not infected.

****

56   *I HAVE SICKE CELL; WILL MY BABY HAVE IT TOO?*

According to the Centre for Disease Control (CDC), People who inherit one sickle cell gene and one normal gene have sickle cell trait and these people usually do not have any of the symptoms of sickle cell disease, but they can pass the trait on to their children.

If both parents have Sickle Cell Trait, there is a 50% (or 1 in 2) chance that any child of theirs also will have Sickle Cell Trait, if the child inherits the sickle cell gene from one of the parents. Such children will not have symptoms of Sickle Cell Disease, but they can pass Sickle Cell Trait on to their children.

If both parents have Sickle Cell Trait, there is a 25% (or 1 in 4) chance that any child of theirs will have Sickle Cell Disease. There is the same 25% (or 1 in 4) chance that the child will not have Sickle Cell Disease or Sickle Cell Trait.

It is therefore very important for a couple to undergo Sickle Cell Disease screening and counselling before a decision to have a child.

****

57 WILL MY PREGNANCY BE AFFECTED BY THE SICKLE CELL DISEASE I HAVE?

It is estimated that at least 35% of pregnancies are complicated by sickle cell crises, and about four- to sixfold of the pregnancies may end up in still births or reduced growth of the babies in the womb Nelson-Piercy (2006).

The Sicked Red Blood Cells usually carry less oxygen and the baby in the womb receives very little of it. This increases the risk of a miscarriage, pre-term labour or even death of the unborn baby in the womb. This is worsened in the time of a crisis as more oxygen is prevented from reaching the unborn baby.

It is therefore recommended that a pregnant woman with sickle cell avoid situations that may trigger a crisis. These includes; exposure to low oxygen environments, dehydration, infections and coldness. Such women need to keep rehydrated and keep warm at all times.

****

<table><tr><td>

58

</td><td>

I AM RHESUS D NEGATIVE; WILL I CARRY MY PREGNANCY TO TERM?

</td></tr></table>

Knowing your blood group as a pregnant woman is very important as this is the basis for transfusing blood in case an emergence arises which may require blood transfusion.

In addition to this Rhesus factor screening is important as it helps to detect possible anti body - antigen reaction known as isoimmunisation which may lead to a miscarriage. This may happen in an event the Rhesus D positive blood of the baby is exposed to the Rhesus D negative one in the mothers' blood stream.

The baby is regarded as a foreign body and antibodies are produced to fight it and may harm the baby.

In such an instance you are advised to get anti-D injection which neutralises the Rhesus D positive antigens that may have entered the mothers blood stream and prevent the reaction and harm that could occur to your baby

****

59   *CAN DIABETES MELLITUS AFFECT MY PREGNANCY?*

Both type 1 and type 2 diabetes mellitus can be complicated by changes that occur in the body because of pregnancy.

There are many risks related to diabetes that can affect both the mother and the unborn baby and these include; very big babies; a condition called macrosomia and this usually lead to a baby being stuck at the shoulders after the head is delivered. The other risks include, miscarriage, congenital malformations, still births and the baby may die immediately after birth.

Good control diabetes before and early in pregnancy can help reduce the risks of miscarriage, congenital malformation, stillbirth and neonatal death, as can folic acid supplements (5 mg/day, taken preconception and up to 12 weeks' gestation).

Weight control is important and women with a Body Mass Index BMI of over 27 kg/m2 are encouraged to lose weight.

It is also highly recommended that you deliver from the hospital with advanced obstetric care.

****

60

MY SUGAR LEVEL HAVE GONE UP, IS RELATED TO PREGNANCY?

Yes it may be related to pregnancy. Diabetes may develop during the pregnancy ans is referred to as gestational diabetes mellitus when it occurs during pregnancy.

The glucose tolerance test is may even be normal except in times of stress, when there may be signs of diabetes. It is however very much associated with history of diabetes in first-degree relatives, previous gestational diabetes, previous baby weighing more than 4.5 kg.

Monitoring your weight and sugar levels is very much recommended if you have any of the above predisposing factors.

> "Babies are always more trouble than you thought—and more wonderful." — Charles Osgood

****

61

CAN I CONTINUE WITH MY DIABETES MELLITUS MEDICATION?

It is important to ensure that as soon as know you are pregnant, you visit your physician to ensure your medications are reviewed. There are some that are recommended and some that are not during pregnancy.

You should also take not that insulin requirements may be increased hence need for adjustment to suit the increased energy demand and consequent insulin need. Rapid acting insulin (aspart and lispro) are considered safe in pregnancy, and of the long-acting insulin, isophane is recommended (NICE 2008b).

Oral diabetes medications other than metformin are not considered safe in pregnancy. If you were taking glibenclamide you therefore need to switch to a drug that is recommended in pregnancy after consultation from your physician.

It is also recommended that monitoring of your sugar levels are enhanced during pregnancy.

****

62 *I HAVE A HEART DISEASE; WILL MY PREGNANCY AFFECT MY CONDITION?*

A pregnant woman with a heart disease may experience more severe symptoms during this period because of the changes that happen in the body and in blood system during pregnancy.

The fluid volume of blood during pregnancy increases by 50% initially and the cellular component increase by 30%. This leads to high volume of blood being taken to the heart hence the heart which has pre-existing condition may be strained.

The risk is even higher in labour when extra blood is shunt from the contracting uterus.

If the heart is failing to pump adequate blood to the uterus because of any condition like heart disease, It may lead to other risks like reduced oxygen delivered to the unborn baby or even death of the baby in the uterus.

The delivery should take place at the hospital with specialized staff and adequate advanced equipment

****

63   *WHY AM I HAVING BLOOD PRESSURE NOW?*

There may be a couple of reasons why your blood pressure may rise during pregnancy. Pregnancy related changes in the body systems most likely the increase in the blood volume can cause that but if you have pre-existing hypertension it may just be triggered or complicated by pregnancy. To help in determining that it is important to not the period when your hypertension sets in.

Hypertension that is related to pregnancy referred to as gestational hypertension usually sets in after 20 weeks in pregnancy and the one that was pre-existing usually become pronounced in the early weeks before your pregnancy is 20 weeks.

Your midwife or physician at your local clinic may check out other things like proteins in urine that may indicate whether this hypertension has complicated into other conditions that increases the risk of losing the unborn baby or the mother.

64

I HAVE ASTHMA; WILL IT AFFECT MY UNBORN BABY OR COMPLICATE MY PREGNANCY?

Asthmatic attacks may be life threatening and are associated with poor pregnancy outcome such as miscarriages and low birth weights as the amount of oxygen delivered to the unborn baby is drastically reduced during an attack.

Asthmatic attacks are caused by the narrowing of the airways and inflammation usually as a response following an exposure to allergens such as pollen, animals, house dust, mites, certain foods, medicines, foods such as dairy products, orange juice, environmental factors, such as dust, chemicals, cigarette smoke, perfumes , exercise, cold or dry air or emotional responses, such as laughing or crying .

However a pregnant woman may experience fewer asthmatic attacks, possibly because of the corticosteroid levels that rise during in pregnancy. Pregnant women however needs to ensure that the above mentioned triggers of an attack are avoided

****

65 ARE THE ASTHMA DRUGS SAFE IN PREGNANCY?

Steroid and anti-inflammatory drugs such as prednisone and hydrocortisone often given by inhalation are safe in pregnancy. They should however be used with caution especially in a pregnant woman with diabetes as well as they increases the sugar levels as well.

These drugs are recommended to control attacks as poorly controlled asthma carries greater risks for the unborn baby than do the drugs used to treat the attack.

Aminophylline should never be used in the control of Asthma in pregnancy except when the benefits outweigh the risks.

> "A baby is God's opinion that life should go on." — Carl Sandburg

****

66 THERE ARE TWIN IN MY FAMILY LINE, AM I POSSIBLY EXPECTING TWINS?

There are two main types of twins and each type occurs in particular circumstances.

Identical twins usually arise when a fertilized egg (zygote) divides into two identical halves during the first 14 days after fertilization. They will have the same genetic make-up and will therefore be of the same sex (Perlman et al 1990). This twinning is highly associated with the use of fertility drugs.

Fraternal twins result from the fertilization of two separate ova (eggs) by two separate sperm. They may be of the same or of different sex and are no more genetically alike than any other siblings. This twining is the one that is associated with a gene that promote hyperovulation or releasing of more than one over in a single month is is passed from a mother to a daughter.

You are therefore only likely to have hereditary twins if your mother line or sister has history of twins.

67

I HAVE EPILEPSY, CAN THAT AFFECT MY PREGNANCY?

Frequent epileptic attacks may affect your unborn baby as the baby receives very little oxygen during a seizure. There may growth retardation and the baby may suddenly die during a seizure.

Seizures may be triggered when women are stressed, tired, in pain, or in hot and steamy environments, and women should be advised about this (Billington & Stevenson 2007).

Sometimes seizures may occur in rapid succession resulting in a condition known as status epilepticus which is uncommon but very serious. It is there important that pregnant women with epilepsy avoid the triggers and also ensure that the condition is under control this period.

> "A new baby is like the beginning of all things – wonder, hope, a dream of possibilities." — Eda LeShan

68 CAN I STILL TAKE ANTI-EPILEPTIC DRUGS?

There are several drugs that are used to control epilepsy. These include; phenytoin sodium, Phenobarbital, carbamezapine and sodium valproate but all of them have a potential to harm pregnancy especially when a combination of them is used and the effect may be worse in the first 3 months when the parts of the unborn baby are being formed.

It is therefore recommended that only one type of drug is used in pregnancy and Carbamezapine has be seen to have less side effects.

first trimester, and throughout pregnancy for women taking sodium valproate. For the same reason, clotting factors may be inhibited in both mother and baby.

> "Words cannot express the joy of new life." — Hermann Hesse

****

69 *I HAVE A FEVER; CAN THAT AFFECT MY PREGNANCY?*

Mild fever for a short period of time is usually not something a pregnant woman should be concerned with. It has however been observed that very high fever for prolonged periods may increase the heart rate of the unborn baby and that may lead to insufficient delivery of oxygen to the tissues.

Sustained High fevers may also lead to a miscarriage of premature labour.

Any cause of fever should be attended to as soon as possible. These may include urinary tract infection

****

70

HAVE I GAINED TOO MUCH WEIGT? HOW MUCH SHOULD I GAIN IN PREGNANCY?

The recommended weight a pregnant woman should have is around 12.5 kg. Appropriate weight gain usually result in the right birth weight of the baby.

On the other hand being overweight in pregnancy comes with a lot of complicatlons including hypertension and diabetes related to pregnancy.

The Confidential Enquiry into Maternal and Child Health 2003– 2005 found that almost 30% of women who had a stillbirth or neonatal death were clinically obese, while 35% had a body mass index of 30 or above (Lewis 2007).

Maternal obesity is associated with an increased risk of gestational diabetes, hypertension and pre-eclampsia (Dixit & Girling 2008)

> "Feeling fat lasts nine months but the joy of becoming a mom lasts forever." – **Nikki Dalton**

71 WHEN IS IT SAFE TO DO AN ULTRA SOUND SCAN?

An ultra sound can be done at any point in pregnancy even at the earliest possible time. As a midwife I actually recommend to my clients that a routine Ultra sound is done at least three times in pregnancy. The first scan which is recommended in the first three months may actually help to confirm pregnancy and probably the age of the pregnancy. The first ultra Sound Scan is very much recommended between weeks 1 to 14 in pregnancy.

The second scan may be done between 14 and 17 weeks after the basic baby parts are formed. Formation of much of baby parts happens during this period. Ultra Sound scans are also recommended after 18 weeks to ascertain the function of the newly formed parts in the womb. The third and final scan may also be used to ascertain the position of the baby. After 32 weeks in pregnancy the baby is not likely change position. This may help in planning the delivery method of the baby.

72 CAN I TAKE AN X-RAY WHILE I AM PREGNANT?

An X-ray taken early in pregnancy may be harmful especially in the first 3 months of pregnancy when foetal parts are forming. Abdominal exposure to heavy dose x-rays in the early weeks of pregnancy is highly associated with birth defects, intellectual disabilities and growth restrictions.

If you suspect you're pregnant you need to avoid exposure to x-rays or radiation. You need to inform your physician if it has been ordered for any investigation.

It can however be done later in pregnancy if the benefits outweigh the risks with little chance of harming the baby when the pregnancy is advanced.

> "The amazing thing about becoming a parent is that you will never again be your own first priority." — Olivia Wilde

73. WHEN CAN I KNOW THE SEX OF MY UNBORN BABY?

Unlike our ancestors and forefathers who depended on dreams and superstition to tell the sex of the unborn baby, modern technology allows you to know the sex of your unborn baby months before you actually give birth.

An ultrasound scan can pick the sex of your unborn baby just 18 weeks after conceptions. If you have 3 scheduled scans in the course of your pregnancy, the second scan can be scheduled around 18 -20 weeks if you have included knowing the sex of your baby as one of the reason for taking a scan.

> "A baby is a wishing well. Everyone puts their hopes, their fears, their pasts, their two cents in." — Elizabeth Bard

****

74

I DELIVERED BY CAESAREAN SECTION, WILL THAT BE THE CASE THIS TIME AGAIN?

Comprehensive history is taken during your very first antenatal visit you make to your health facility. Among the details that we get is history of your past surgical operations including caesarean sections that were done previously. The reason for the operations done is reviewed to determine what could have led to the operation.

A physical examination, particularly of your pelvis will then be done at your local clinic to assess if a normal delivery can be possible for you.

A combination of both your past history and physical examination will help to tell. If the reasons of your previous C-section were related to the physical aspect that could not change then a normal delivery may not be possible again.

However it is not always that when you delivered by C-section you'll always deliver that way. Perhaps the baby didn't just turn and this time the baby may turn on its own.

****

75 — *WHEN SHOULD I START VISITING ANTENATAL CLINIC?*

The purpose of antenatal care is to improve and maintain maternal and foetal health by monitoring the progress of pregnancy to confirm normality and detect any deviation early so that corrective care can be provided.

The formation of the baby parts also happens in the very first weeks of pregnancy and there are several things a pregnant woman should know just at that particular time for instance medications to avoid.

Pregnant women actually experience a lot of physical and emotional challenges at this particular time and a midwife should just come in at this particular time.

It is therefore recommended that women start antenatal care as soon as they confirm that they are pregnant. This will enable them access optimum care as early as possible.

Knowledge of danger signs should also be obtained as early as possible so that appropriate care may be sought and rendered in an event one occurs.

****

76

HOW OFTEN SHOULD I VISIT THE ANTENATAL CLINIC FOR ROUTINE CHECK UP?

To ensure that both quality and outcomes of the pregnancy are enhanced, a pregnant woman needs to visit the health care worker for appropriate information, physical check up, prevention and treatment of any abnormalities that may exist during pregnancy. To ensure this is achieved, antenatal care visits are scheduled systematically according to the needs of the mother and the unborn baby.

The World Health Organisation (WHO) recommends that a pregnant woman should have at least 8 times contacts with a Health Care provider rather than just a visit to a health facility during pregnancy.

The first contact is recommended as soon as pregnancy is confirmed and before 12 weeks. The second visit is recommended at 20 weeks, the third visit at 26 weeks, and the fourth visit at 30 weeks. The fifth one is done at 34 weeks, the sixth at 36 weeks, the seventh at 38 weeks and the 8th visit is done at 40 weeks.

****

Each visit is aligned with particular objectives that are met towards the goal of improving the outcome of the pregnancy.

The wellbeing of both the mother and the unborn baby are checked at every single visit the mother makes to the facility and has contact with a professional health care provider.

> "We can't understand when we're pregnant, or when our siblings are expecting, how profound it is to have a shared history with a younger generation: blood, genes, humor. It means we were actually here, on Earth, for a time—like the Egyptians with their pyramids, only with children." —

****

77

I FEEL OKAY, IS ANTENATALCARE STILL NECESSARY?

Antenatal Care is still very important because it doesn't just look at the now when you are fine but prepare you to handle every single day of the 280 you are expected to carry your unborn baby During this period, you and your family will be prepared for the physical, psychological and emotional adaptation to handle pregnancy as well as for safe birth. You will be helped by a skilled Health care worker to draw an appropriate birth plan to facilitate a fulfilling experience for you. During this period, health care workers will equip you with knowledge of aspects essential for childbirth and for early parenthood. Infant feeding methods and counselling to prepare you for lactation and feeding of your baby will be provided to you by health care professionals.

Health Care workers will also help you to know how to identify danger signs and how to promptly respond to them so that the outcome of your pregnancy is the positive one.

****

78   *WHY SHOULD I TAKE VITAMIN SUPPLEMENTATION?*

Nutrients and vitamins are very important during pregnancy as early as the conception period. Nutrients provide building blocks for the development of a newly conceived baby.

As much as there may be an assurance the pregnant woman is taking right nutrients and vitamins from the daily intake. It should be understood that risking a deficiency of any may lead to disastrous results. For instance a deficiency of folate may lead to major deformities in the baby.

Therefore supplementation of vitamins is highly recommended prior conceiving and during pregnancy.

In addition to this, there is an increased demand of energy for both the mother and the developing unborn baby.

****

79

IS IT POSSIBLE TO TELL I WILL DELIVER NORMALLY?

Yes it is possible to tell whether you will deliver normally through the physical examinations and use of modern technology.

A midwife or a clinician may conduct physical examination on your abdomen and pelvis to determine how your baby is positions in the womb. Detailed examination of how adequate your pelvis is to allow the baby to pass through may also be done.

An ultrasound scan is also very recommended as it reveals the size of your baby and how positioned your baby is.

Based on the above assessments, a midwife or physician may then help you to plan for your delivery and advise on the possible method of delivery.

****

80 *WHY AM I SO ANXIOUS?*

The hormonal and physical changes that occur during pregnancy easily predispose pregnant woman to anxiety and possible depression. Pregnant women worry about the outcome of the pregnancy, the health of their unborn baby, the financial requirements and sometimes the physical chances that pregnancy brings. Women may also stress on how they will take care of their baby.

This anxiety is even worse according to observations for women who have had experienced miscarriages or had a caesarean section due to any obstetric abnormality in their previous pregnancies.

It is however that this anxiety is attended as soon as possible to avoid negative effects especially during labour. Post delivery this may culminate into a serious depression or mental illness known as Puerperal Psychosis.

****

81   *WILL THIS ANXIETY AFFECT LABOUR?*

Yes it will definitely affect the progress of labour which may lead to an undesired outcome.

Your body produce a lot of adrenaline when you're are anxious, this adrenaline will counteract a chemical in the body called Oxytocin which is responsible for ensuring that the way is opening and the muscles gain enough power to push your baby out.

Anxiety will therefore slow down the process of labour and the unborn baby may be distressed in the process. That is why as I midwife I will tell you that your personality in labour is as important as the force that you need to push the baby out.

Ensure that your relationship with healthcare personnel is built and you acquaint yourself to the environment where you will deliver from. Family members should also be available to support the woman and reduce stress in return.

****

82   *HOW WILL I TELL IT'S TIME TO DELIVER MY BABY?*

Women have different experiences signifying the onset of child birth. However, there are common experiences that are regarded as signs of child birth.

Two weeks prior to delivery, many women see their abdomen sinking down a bit. This usually signifies the beginning of entry of the head into the birth canal.

Backache and abdominal pains become severe and consistent like a belt being tightened. Women frequently experience abdominal pain months or weeks leading to delivery but when labour starts the intensity is higher.

The plug of mucus that seals the way is dislodged a woman may see a mixture of blood and mucus coming out.

The bag of waters which envelops the baby breaks as the way opens wider and wider in readiness for the baby to come out.

****

83   *CAN I STILL TRAVEL OR DRIVE WHILE I AM PREGNANT?*

Many things change when a woman becomes pregnant. These changes occur due to the changes that occur in the hormone profile in a pregnant woman's body. This affects almost every system in the body.

A pregnant woman will therefore need much rest during this period to save energy as there is a surge in the energy demand during pregnancy. Activities during pregnancy should therefore be modified. Strenuous activities may cause both strain and risk of injury to the unborn baby as well. Activities were trauma is eminent should be avoided as some traumas may lead to premature separation of the placenta while the baby is in the womb and result in a miscarriage. Long hours of travel as well as driving should if possible be avoided in pregnancy. Pregnant women should only take essential travels before 32 weeks in pregnancy. Some airlines and transport companies actually do not carry pregnant women above 32 weeks in pregnancy.

The risk of travelling for long hours may include clotting of blood in the veins especially at the back of the leg; a condition known as deep vein thrombosis. This may later lead to a heart attack or stroke in the brain in an event the clot dislodges and travel to these organs.

Where travel or driving is essential and cannot be avoided, a pregnant woman should learn how to correctly use a seatbelts, including the correct positioning of the seatbelt above and below the womb.

"Motherhood is the biggest gamble in the world. It is the glorious life force. It's huge and scary—it's an act of infinite optimism." – Gilda Radner

84 CAN I TAKE PAIN KILLER IN LABOUR?

Before considering use of analgesia

or any forms of painkiller in labour, you need to understand how each form of pain relief will affect you and your unborn baby.

There is evidence to suggest that epidurals relieve pain, but can increase the numbers of instrumental births and run the risk of causing hypotension, hindering leg movement, fever and urine retention (Jones et al. 2012).

A summary of the evidence from Cochrane Systematic Reviews suggests that non-pharmacological methods such as: immersion in water, relaxation and massage may improve management of labour pain, with few adverse effects, although their efficacy is unclear (Jones et al. 2012).

There is need to weigh the advantages and disadvantages before deciding to use and not use analgesia in labour is considered

85 WHY DO I HAVE A THIS SURGE OF ENERGY..AM NEARING CHILD BIRTH

Women experience a flurry of energy just prior to their delivery a phenomenon commonly known as 'Nesting'. During this time pregnant women tend to clean their houses, rearrange their homes and prepare meals. This usually prepares a women's environment post delivery.

This surge in energy is usually associated with the increase in the oestrogen levels after progesterone begin to fall as pregnancy nears delivery.

86 *SHOULD I BE TALKING TO*

"Babies are bits of star-dust blown from the hand of God. Lucky is the woman who knows the pangs of birth for she has held a star." – *Larry Barretto*

MY UNBORN BABY?

****

Parent baby bonding normally starts way before the baby is born. It is encouraged that a mothers or fathers talk to their unborn babies at least in the 9th month of pregnancy.

The brain of your unborn baby at this stage is wired with an estimated 100 billion neurons. Four weeks away from delivery, evidence shows that these neurons are stimulated and connections are done right at that time about 36 weeks in pregnancy. This is usually triggered by sounds from the outside environment. It is also believed that at this stage the eyes of the unborn baby are open and the unborn baby is able to perceive light from the outside environment.

87 HOW VULNERABLE AM I TO ILLNESSES?

It is believed that the immune

****

system of a woman is suppressed during pregnancy and this works somehow to an advantage to prevent the body from rejecting the newly conceived baby. However a woman becomes vulnerable to other illnesses especially in the first 12 weeks of pregnancy.

The rising levels of corticosteroids in the body in pregnancy are also linked to this suppression in immunity and vulnerability to infections.

It is therefore recommended that pregnant women take preventive measures against contracting infection. These include ensuring drinking water is safe, proper nutrition and mild exercises among other.

88   *WHY AM I VULNERABLE TO VAGINAL INFECTIONS?*

The hormonal changes that occurs during pregnancy changes the PH in the vagina from an acid media to almost neutral and this disturbs the natural barrier against infections. The acid media prevent the thriving of harmful bacteria and viruses.

The diminishing of this natural barrier predisposes the pregnant woman to especially fungal infections the commonest being candidiasis.

Pregnant women are therefore discouraged from using antibacterial or medicated soaps to wash their private parts. Douching is also not encouraged to avoid worsening this condition.

It is therefore recommended that proper screening is done to ensure appropriate treatment may be given if a pregnant woman present with either foul smelling discharge or anything unusual from the private part.

****

89 *HOW CAN I KNOW THIS DISCHARGE IS NORMAL OR ABNORMAL?*

Normal discharge which is slightly increased in pregnancy is white non offensive and is not accompanied by itching or pain when passing urine.

Abnormal discharges as a infections can also be identified by their characteristic features when they occur in pregnancy.

Trichomoniasis is a common sexually transmitted infection that produces a discharge but this one is usually frothy yellowish and is accompanied by itching and pain on passing urine.

Chlamydia is another sexually transmitted infection which produces a discharge but this one also can be differentiated by its puss like discharge sometimes mixed with blood.

Gonorrhoea also produces discharges that looks like pass and is usually accompanied by pain on passing urine.

Candidiasis which is the commonest produces a white cardy discharge accompanied by itching.

****

90 *HOW LONG DOES PREGNANCY LAST?*

Pregnancy lasts for 280 days from conceptions or 40 weeks. This doesn't mean your delivery will take place at day number 280. Several factors determine the onset of labour; it may come earlier than that, sometimes as early as week 37 or after 40 weeks depending on the conditions.

It has been noted that labour frequently start early in multiple pregnancies and this has been associated by the over stretching of the uterus.

> "Rigid plans work best if you're building a skyscraper; with something as mysteriously human as giving birth, it's best, both literally and figuratively, to keep your knees bent." — Mark Sloan

91 HOW SAFE IS IT TO DELIVER FROM HOME?

A good number of home deliveries are still being recorded especially from the developing countries. This has however been seen as one of the contributing factors to the high maternal deaths that are recorded in developing countries.

Delivering at home in the absence of skilled health care workers and equipment used for monitoring the progress of labour or any complication that may arise during this period may be very risky which is not very encouraged.

A delivery is considered safe when it happen in the health facility in the presence of a Skilled Health Care Worker.

Delivering from home may predispose a woman to not only complications but post delivery infections since the environment may not be as the hospital environment where infection prevention is done with the techniques of based on science and research.

92   *I HAD A MISCARIAGE PREVIOUSLY, ARE THERE CHANCES IT MAY RECUR?*

It is very hard to tell whether your current pregnancy will end up in a miscarriage based on your previous experience as a number of factors need to be reviewed to determine this.

The cause of your previous miscarriage need to be evaluate; If your miscarriage was caused for instance by incompatibility of your Rhesus factor it may likely recur if you don't receive anti D injection. If it is as a result of an incompetent cervix, it may recur if no interventions are taken.

It should however be noted that if the cause was a once off incidence like a bout of untreated malaria or syphilis. It is unlikely to happen if the underlying cause which affected the pregnancy is not present.

****

93   *WITH SO MUCH CHANGE, HOW LONG WILL IT TAKE TO RETURN TO NORMAL?*

Hormones cause so much change in all the systems in the body during pregnancy. As pregnancy nears the end and delivery approaches, hormone supply declines including from the placenta that is removed immediately after you give birth.

This process takes a woman back to near normal in a period of 6 weeks after delivering. The concentration of blood goes back to normal and as hormones clear from the body the systems goes back to normal as well.

The skin pigments clears, weight steadily reduces, muscles which were softened begin to tone up back to their normal state. Heart burn resolves and many other changes that took place begin to reverse.

It is recommended that a woman take mild exercises, plenty of fluids and proteins during this period to aid healing and return to normal.

****

94 — *WHAT WILL BE THE FIRST THING I WILL BE EXPECTED TO DO AFTER DELIVERING?*

You will be expected to put the baby to your breast at least within that very hour you will deliver your baby. This practice has so many benefits to your baby.

The first breast milk in this period provides a passive immunity against diseases that the baby receives from the mother.

It also provides the energy resources that the baby needs as they start a new life outside the mother's womb.

This process also helps the mother to start bonding with their newborn baby.

> "A new baby is like the beginning of all things—wonders, hope, and dream of possibilities." — Eda J. LeShan

****

95

HOW WILL I ENSURE I HAVE BREAST MILK TO GIVE TO MY BABY FROM DAY ONE?

During pregnancy your body begins to prepare for the immediate tasks that you will be required to perform immediately after delivery.

Early in pregnancy the glands that produce breast milk begin to prepare in order to carry out this function normally. Milk production is almost guaranteed immediately you deliver your baby as a result of these processes. Compassion and desire to breast feed your baby also increase the production.

More milk is produced immediately the baby suckles from the breast. The key ensure sustained production is to ensure milk glands are emptied every time to promote flow. The mother needs to ensure that she is well hydrated enough flow.

****

96 *HOW WELL CAN I PREPARE FOR PREGNANCY?*

Preparations for pregnancy are important and immediately you contemplate pregnancy, preparations should start.

It is recommended that a woman takes 0.4 mg of folic acid everyday 3 months before becoming pregnant to ensure the baby is formation is without defects as part of the preparations. You also need to ensure that you are fully vaccinated against tetanus.

Social habits such as smoking and alcohol drinking should be modified as these may also interfere with the formation of the baby.

If you have been working in environments where there are chemicals, you need to consider a break during this critical moment. Exposure to substances like lead may have devastating effects.

You also need to ensure that both you and your partner are screened from genetic diseases such as sickle cell disease as well as blood types including rhesus compatibilities.

It is also recommended the adequate nutrition and an appropriate are attained.

****

97 *HOW WELL CAN I PREPARE FOR LABOR AND DELIVERY?*

Preparation for labour should start as early as possible and you need to prepare yourself both psychologically and physically to ensure a positive outcome is achieved.

Psychological state of a woman in labour in labour is one of the 4 P's among them Powers and Passage (birth canal and Passenger (Size of the baby) that determine whether the progress and outcome of labour will be positive.

Inability to prepare psychologically may hinder progress of labour in that the chemicals that are produced in anxiety blocks the action of hormones that facilitate the opening of the way.

Physical preparations which include, learning breathing techniques which ensure maximum oxygen is delivered to your unborn baby at the time supply of blood reduced as labour intensifies.

Adequate hydration to ensure muscle contraction which generates the power that pushes the baby out is not hindered. A diet high in calories to ensure energy reserves for muscles contraction is replenished.

98 — *WHAT ARE THE MUST HAVE CONTACTS IN MY PHONE BOOK?*

A pregnant woman needs to have contact lines for certain service providers that should be available to her 24 hours a day to ensure readiness for emergencies and delivery.

At all times from the very early stages of pregnancy, transport should be readily available and within reach regardless of time, you and your family can pre-arrange for that.

You need to ensure that you stay constantly in touch your midwife or doctor you can reach anytime during the day and in the night. In cases where your community has Safe Motherhood agent, you need to ensure that you have their contact lines as well.

Your key family members that are supposed to play a role in ensuring you get to the health facility need to ready all the time and their contact lines open 24 hours day.

****

99   *HOW MANY HOURS WILL I BE EXPECTED TO LABOUR?*

After waiting for 280 long days I know you wouldn't love to wait much longer for you to meet this miracle growing big and round under your skin.

Labour is the closing moment of this long period of expectation, uncertainty, anxiety, hope and optimism. It is also a door to a new world of motherhood with a whole new set of roles and responsibilities but for how long will you wait once this labour begins.

Labour last for an average of 6 hours for a woman who has delivered birth before and about 8 hours for someone who has never given birth before; this can be more or less depending on how favourable the conditions may be.

It should however be noted that labour lasting for more than 12 hours is delayed and if you attempted to deliver from home engage a midwife or doctor immediately.

****

100 IAM PACKING MY BAG FOR LABOUR WHAT DO I INCLUDE?

Among the many things you are considering to pack in your maternity bag ensure that the limited space doesn't make you forget to pack the most essential and these should include;

For mommy

1. Maternity Clothes – To go home in
2. Nursing Bra- To allow breast milk flow
3. Maternity pads – to catch the post delivery flow
4. Snacks and water- remember you need energy and hydration for labour.
5. Hand sanitizer – for your hand hygiene

For baby

1. Baby layette – this includes blanket, sweater, head dress, socks, showel and going home outfit
2. Wipes

Others

1. Camera and lenses- remember you need to keep the first moments memorable
2. Contact list to share the news with.

****

References

1. Drake P. 2016, *Cigarette Smoking during Pregnancy*, Centre for Disease Control, New York.

2. Lewis L, 2015, *Fundamentals of Midwifery; A textbook for students*, first edition, Wiley-Blackwell, West Sussex.

3. Macdonald, S and Magill-Cuerden, J, 2010, *Mayes' Midwifery,* Fourteenth edition, Elsevier, London.

4. Sellers P, M, 1993, *Midwifery, a textbook and reference book for midwives in Southern Africa*, Volume One, Juta and Company, Cape Town.

5. Walsh, D and Downe, S, 2010, *Essential Midwifery Practice: Intra partum Care*, first edition, Wiley-Blackwell, West Sussex.

6. WHO, *Recommendation on antenatal care for a Positive pregnancy experience*, 2016, Geneva